Dementia:

How Will Dementia Affect My life? Diagnosis and Treatment

Dr. David Carter

or otherwise, by any usage or abuse of any policies, processes, or directions contained within is the solitary and utter responsibility of the recipient reader. Under no circumstances will any legal responsibility or blame be held against the publisher for any reparation, damages, or monetary loss due to the information herein, either directly or indirectly.

The information herein is offered for informational purposes solely, and is universal as so. The presentation of the information is without contract or any type of guarantee assurance.

Table of Contents

Introduction

I want to thank and congratulate you for downloading the book, *"Dementia: How Will Dementia Affect My Life? Diagnosis and Treatment"*.

This book contains proven steps and strategies on how to better understand and treat dementia. Dementia is a common condition that affects the older population, as well as a condition that creates many different problems associated with this disease. It can often take a toll on the body as well as the relationships one has with others. Losing your memory can be very disturbing, and for many, it can be a tragic realization of one's mortality.

This book was written to help in your understanding of this condition, allowing you to assess any associated risk factors. Dementia is certainly a problematic sort of occurrence, and for those that have an affected family member, it can be disheartening. Don't let it throw you or others into despair. This book will allow you to comprehend and gain an understanding so that you can handle the disease's progression, in the hopes of helping those affected, either directly or indirectly. Education is the key to understanding and hopefully overcoming.

Chapter 1: What is Dementia?

The first key is to understand the different components that make up the term dementia. It's not just memory loss; it encompasses so much more. This chapter will discuss what dementia is, and what you can do about it.

Dementia is not one type of disease. It's a kind of condition that has a wide array of symptoms attached to it. However, the major one noticed in all of them is the loss of memory and thinking skills. Typically, this is severe enough to stop a person from the ability to perform daily activities.

For many people, this means that often, their family members might not remember who they are. It often results in losing the ability to move as well. Alzheimer's is the first thing that usually comes to mind when one thinks of the term dementia. We will address this in Chapter 2. Vascular dementia often presents after a stroke and is the second most common type. However, many other different conditions can be the cause; some of them reversible. Thyroid issues and vitamin deficiencies are often reversible conditions. However, memory loss often increases over time.

Dementia is often regarded as senility or being senile, but that's a misconception. We are not referring to the ordinary mental decline noticed with aging. It presents as a severe loss of memory and different from what your typical senility and the effects of aging can do to a human being.

With dementia, often the person that's afflicted can't go out and perform their regular daily routine. They've soon degenerated to the point where they struggle to move about, which results in the need for someone to assist them and the loss of their independence. The family becomes the primary caregiver, however, many times a family will choose the option of seeking the assistance of nursing homes or assisted living facilities. Dementia often progresses to the point where the patient loses any memory of their family and friends. It's a condition that if often hard to cope. Many have to deal with the ones they love falling into a bottomless pit in which there appears no way out.

In essence, dementia is the loss of the mental facility. It's a severe condition, but this chapter gave you an oversight as to what it is, and these following sections will go into the

Dementia

types, causes, treatment, and prevention of dementia.

Chapter 2: Dealing with Dementia in everyday life

Being a dementia patient, caring a friend or family member with dementia poses numerous difficulties for families and guardians. Whoever with dementia conditions, for example, Alzheimer's and related illnesses have a progressive genetic mind issue or disorder that makes it more difficult for them to recall things, think clearly, speak with others, or deal with themselves. What's more, dementia can bring about emotional episodes and even change a man's identity and conduct.

Communications difficulties can be a be notable amongst the most disturbing parts of nurturing to someone with Alzheimer's or some other kind of dementia — and it's baffling for those with the disease and for friends and family.

Despite the fact that it can be difficult to understand why individuals with dementia act the way they do, the clarification is unsettled to their disease and the progressions it causes in the brain.

Acquaint yourself with a common situation that you may encounter when somebody has dementia, so that if your adored one says something shocking, you'll know how to react smoothly and effectively.

People are not born knowing how to deal with a man with dementia—yet we can learn. Enhancing your relational abilities will make care giving less stressful and will probably enhance the nature of your relationship with your loved one. Great relational abilities will likewise improve your capacity to handle the difficult conduct you may experience as you watch over a man with a twisting illness.

You may already know about changes in your capability to finish day by day assignments that once easily fell into place for you. Whether you are the patient of dementia or just a care taker; this book will help you a lot. Building up your own coping systems doesn't need to be annoying. You can reorganize the procedure by concentrating on these simple tips. Here are some helpful tips to respond effectively when dealing with dementia in your everyday life;

Start up a good relationship when interacting

When you are going to deal with a person with dementia, you should get his/her attention carefully. Simply turning off the TV or radio is very helpful so they can focus on what you are saying. Before talking, ensure you have her attention; address her by name, recognize yourself by name and connection, and use nonverbal signs and touch to keep her focused. Your attitude and non-verbal gestures tell your emotions and thoughts stronger than your words. Set a positive personality by addressing your cherished one in a lovely and conscious way. Use facial expression, manner of speaking and physical touch to deliver your message and show your feelings of concern.

Use straightforward words and sentences. Talk slowly, clearly and in a calming tone. If ever that she doesn't comprehend the first time, utilize the same wording, simple and straight to repeat your message or question.

Conduct healthy habits

A person with dementia still needs a quality and enjoyable life; however without some help from families and others, it is a great deal more difficult for them to accomplish their purpose and joy. There are numerous approaches to arrange and give fitting exercises to individuals with dementia. Understanding the individual with dementia will help you to arrange suitable exercises for them. This implies knowing the individual's previous lifestyle, past work, hobbies, leisure and common interests, past travel experience and significant life occasions.

A man with dementia may appreciate a trip, regardless of the fact that they don't recollect where they have been. What is essential is that the moment is appreciated, despite the fact that the experience might be soon unseen.

If your loved one is interested in some kind of physical activities, these are some recommended exercise to try;

Walking – this is one of the best all-round activities, and it's free. Strolling likewise works off the irritable tendency to meander that is run of the mill of Alzheimer's patients. Take a try at consolidating the walk with an important task, for example, going to market to buy something.

Cycling – a two-person bike permits you to sit in front and control the bicycle, while your traveler sits in the secondary lounge and pedals. On the off chance that the individual with dementia has issues with their equalization, you could have a go at employing a three-wheeled bike for them to ride, while you cycle close by them

Gym work outs – for example, treadmills, stationary bikes and weight machines

Dynamic exercise – you could go to classes together to exercise like aerobics.

Always have a good food on the table

Individuals with dementia actually start to forget that they have to eat and drink. The outcomes of poor nutrition are frequent, including weight reduction, irritability, restlessness, bladder or gut issues and confusion.

Always prepare nutritious food for your loved one. In the event that they have dentures or inconvenience biting or swallowing, make sure that all your prepared food is soft and able to eat easily.

If ever that loss of weight is an issue, offer nutritious high – calorie between foods. Breakfast foods high in sugars are regularly favored. Then again, if the issue is weight gain, keep away unhealthy foods r high – calories food. Rather, give them a hand of fresh fruits, veggie plate and other fresh low-calorie snacks.

Maintain pleasant ambiance

Peoples with dementia ought to live in a domain that gives comfort, routines and social opportunities. It ought to be natural and offer significant exercises that the patient appreciates, not ones expected to simply fill the time. Make rooms simple to explore, use simple and relaxing colors, use photographs and music to unwind and lift the soul, have the temperature suit the patient's sensitivities.

Always make sure that the patients have a telephone close

to them at all times and make use a basic stylistic theme to minimize diversions and uncertain dangers. Drive out floor coverings, and introduce snatch bars in the bathroom if needed. Welcome all the guests who wanted to visit. Loved ones can animate recollections and laughers.

Support medical check ups

The individual you are caring of has a mind issue that shapes who he has become. When you attempt to control or change his conduct, you'll in all chances fail or be met with resistance. Check with the specialist first. Behavioral issues may have a hidden therapeutic reason: maybe the individual is in distress or encountering an unfavorable symptom from drugs. Sometimes, similar to incontinence or hallucinations, there might be some medicine or treatment that can help with dealing with the issue.

Individuals with dementia regularly can't let us know what they need or need. They may accomplish something, similar to remove all the clothes from the wardrobe every day, and we ask why. It is likely that the individual is satisfying should be occupied and beneficial.

The way to overseeing difficult practices is being innovative and adaptable in your techniques to address a given issue.

Always have an ear to listen

Individuals with dementia will regularly repeat a word, explanation, inquiry or movement again and again. While this kind of conduct is normally safe for the individual with dementia, it can irritate and unpleasant to guardians. Once in a while the behavior is activated by nervousness, fatigue, dread or natural factors. Avoid advising them that they just asked the same inquiry. Have a go at disregarding the conduct or address, and rather have a go at refocusing the individual into an action.

Get a peaceful sleep

Numerous individuals living with dementia experience difficulty getting the opportunity to rest, or wake up regularly amid the night. Focus on increasing their comfort amid the numerous hours they may spend awake around evening time.

Set Realistic goals

Set reasonable and realistic goals for yourself and utilize the skills you must do in dealing with this challenging disease. A few tasks may turn out to be excessively hard for you, making it impossible to finish even you always have reminder aids. Decrease stress by approaching family or companions for help.

If ever you are a dementia patient or caring a person with dementia who is near you or close to you, your relationship will change extraordinarily over the long haul.

You may likewise encounter feelings of melancholy and loss as the sickness advances. There are such a variety of changes that and routine when looking after somebody with dementia that it can be difficult for care takers to manage their sentiments.

Figuring out how to acknowledge what you can't change may feel truly upsetting, yet it could make life appear to be significantly more acceptable.

When you are the person with dementia, things you once did effectively will turn out to be progressively difficult, for example, keeping up a calendar. Tolerating changes in your capacities and adjusting new adapting skills can help you reestablish harmony to your life and give you a sense of attainment in your capabilities as you keep on fighting and living with the dementia disease.

The more you understand the difficulties that dementia can bring, the better you will have the capacity to adapt for everyday living.

Chapter 3: What Are The Types of Dementia?

One thing to know about dementia is that there are a few major types. These are important to know, because while dementia is the big umbrella these all fall under, some of the other forms of dementia differ from others. This chapter will go into the various types of dementia, what happens to the person, as well as treatment factors.

Alzheimer's

This the most common form of dementia and is responsible for about 60-80% of the cases that come through most clinics. Typically, when you have this, you stop remembering recent conversations as well as names or even events. Memory loss is one of the first clinical symptoms that present. Depression and apathy are also early presenting symptoms. Later, people who suffer from this can exhibit impaired communication, lack of judgment, disorientation, confusion, and difficulties in swallowing, walking, or speaking.

In the brain, there are abnormalities seen on an MRI or brain scan. Typically, this is caused by the presence of beta-amyloid and twisted strands of the protein tau. Often, there is evidence of damage to the nerve cells and even some death of different segments of the brain.

Vascular Dementia

Less common than Alzheimer's, Vascular Dementia encompasses about 10% of cases. This type of dementia typically appears after you suffer a stroke or other significant brain infarct.

The symptoms usually include a lack of judgment and the inability to make important decisions, planning, or organizational skills. Different from Alzheimer's, it affects the decision-making processes, whereas Alzheimer's affects memory loss. The cause is the blockage of blood vessels and damage that led to strokes or brain bleeding. Often, the location of the occurrence, the number of events, and the scope of the brain injury determine how bad the thinking process is affected.

The brain changes can be seen in the blood vessels that is affected. In the past, the evidence for this was used to help a doctor determine if this was vascular dementia or Alzheimer's, but the practice is not consistent because of the pathological changes that often occur. If you have multiple forms of dementia, it will often present itself in different areas of the brain. If there are two or more types, the diagnosis is mixed dementia, a rare but far-reaching occurrence.

Dementia with Lewy Bodies

Dementia with Lewy bodies, categorized with memory loss and cognition impairment, is often seen with Alzheimer's. The difference with this is that with DLB, you suffer from more sleep disturbances, hallucinations, slowness, gait imbalance, and movements similar to Parkinson's. Often, when one suffers from Parkinson's, which is more of an action type of dementia, it's often diagnosed as a form of this kind of dementia.

With Lewy bodies, there is typically an abnormal clumping of a protein called alpha-syncline. When this develops in the cortex, dementia is the result. These proteins can also be in brains of Parkinson's patients, but the aggregates are typically more in a pattern that is different from DLB. The brain changes with DLB can cause dementia or coincide with other forms of dementia, and each of these abnormalities can contribute to the development of various dementia. When you have more than one of these as a diagnosis, mixed dementia occurs, and typically, one of these three will present as the diagnosis.

When you're looking to understand the different types of dementia, often these three are the most talked about, with other forms described as a branch off from these three primary diagnoses. By understanding that, you'll be able to see why the brain does what it does, along with the various elements to dementia that you might not have understood before. Gaining an understanding of these three primary causes of dementia is the key to determining the best course of treatment and how to proceed to get the best outcome for the patient.

Chapter 4: What Causes Dementia?

Dementia has a various amount of causes along with symptoms. By understanding the different aspects of dementia, you'll be able to get a better understanding of the condition and causes.

Dementia caused by brain cell damage interrupts the ability of brain cells to talk to one another. When the brain cells aren't able to communicate correctly, many times the thinking, the various behavior people suffer from, and even feelings can change.

The brain is responsible for many different functions determined by regions of the brain. Some of these areas are responsible for various functions, such as memory, judgment, and movement. When cells in a particular segment of the brain are damaged, the region won't be able to do the functions they were designed to perform.

With dementia, different areas are associated with the various kinds of dementia and the types of brain cell damage. For example, when you talk about Alzheimer's, there are higher levels of individual portions of the brain cells, which make it harder for them to be healthy and even talk to one another. The brain also has this area called the hippocampus, which is the area where learning and memory are in the brain, and the cells within this area are often the first to be damaged when Alzheimer's happens. That's why memory loss and the inability to learn things is one of the most common sorts of things you see in those that suffer from that.

Often, the changes in the brain that cause this only get worse with time, many times the thinking and memory problems that come about are due to other conditions and should be treated individually. These conditions are listed below:

- Depression
- The side effects of medication
- Overuse of alcohol,
- Thyroid issues
- The lack of vitamins and nutrition

These are typically treatable to some degree, but Alzheimer's and other forms of dementia, in general, are not treatable.

Symptoms

When talking about the symptoms, often, one just thinks memory loss. However, there are more than just that, and this section will go over some of the major symptoms associated with that.

When you have these, they can vary in great amounts, but at least two of these must be reduced or impaired to be considered dementia, and they are listed below:

- Language and communication
- The ability to pay attention
- Judgment and decision-making
- Visualizing and perception
- Memory

With those that suffer from dementia, often, they suffer from short term memory issues, such as not being able to keep track of paying bills, planning various activities, appointments, remembering where items are, and even wandering. When it progresses, it starts out slowly and then it gradually gets worse. If you start to notice some memory changes or the inability to remember various things such as thinking and making decisions, the best thing to do is not to ignore them. You should make sure that you or the one suffering does go to the doctor to help you determine what the condition is. When the symptoms do suggest dementia, it's also good because early diagnosis means that the treatment will work better, and there is a chance that they'll be able to remember more things for a longer span of time, which is always good.

With dementia, there are many associated factors. This chapter went over some of the causes and symptoms. Often, this is something that you as a person can watch for, improving your ability to see the issues, and from there, working to benefit from this as well now, and in the future.

Chapter 5: What Are The Treatments For Dementia?

Let's say that you start to suffer from memory loss. You might want to go into the doctor' to see what it is. This chapter will go over the treatment and care of dementia.

Diagnosis

Unfortunately, there isn't one particular test that will tell you if someone has this condition. With many of these circumstances, doctors will diagnose this after they take a look at the medical history, a physical exam, lab test, and even monitoring the changes in your thinking and daily function.

From this, a doctor might also start to look at how he responds to other people in the world. People with dementia respond in different ways to others. If you notice that someone you love is starting to forget you, doctors should address this, and it'll help them determine what course of treatment should be initiated.

Often when it comes to dementia, doctors won't know right away what form of dementia a person has, since it manifests itself in similar ways. Sometimes as well, a person might have mixed symptoms or mixed dementia. However, they will tell you if you have dementia, but they won't tell you what type it is. Once they inform the patient however, they'll send you to a neurologist to help you with further consultation

Treatment

Due to the different forms of dementia, treatment might be different for a patient on a case-by-case basis. Often, because a doctor might not know right away if a person has Alzheimer's or Parkinson's, they might treat dementia as a generalized condition. In that case, they administer drugs to help you with this.

However, it should be known that there isn't a cure for progressive dementia. While there are drugs to slow it down, there isn't a cure-all to stop it. Even with that though, with proper regulation you can keep the condition in check in an effective manner.

Typically, a doctor would choose to prescribe memory medications for early conditions of this. If there is a problem underneath it all, such as alcohol abuse and the like, a doctor might intervene to help with these various issues. If the dementia is coming up because of medication, a doctor might work to switch the medications up. However, often if it's gone for too long, a doctor won't be able to do anything, but these treatments do help slow the progression of the condition.

Often however, if the patient's dementia progresses, they won't be able to live on their own anymore, which is not a fun situation. If it comes down to this, and the person doesn't have a spouse that can assist them, the doctor might ask the family to take care of the patient, or ask for them to be put into a retirement home if not feasible. Often, this is at the discretion of the family members involved.

With dementia, the treatment and prognosis of this is still not completely detailed, but many doctors are still working day in and day out to help a patient that suffers from this condition stick around for a bit longer.

Right now, the path to understanding dementia and finding a cure for it is still a bit foggy, but there is new research and new clinical studies that are being done to help with this. Ultimately, the test of time will tell if there will ever be a cure or not.

Chapter 6: Risks and Preventions You can do

While there isn't a cure for dementia, there are still activities a person can do to help prevent this condition from coming about. Maybe you're a young adult who doesn't want to suffer from this when older. Or maybe, you start to wonder if you're at risk for this condition and you would like to prevent it. There are activities you can implement into your life to help deter this condition, and this chapter will go over what you can do.

You might be reading this because you have someone you love who suffers from this condition. Perhaps you might want to make sure that you're not at risk as well. Maybe you've been exposed to the true nature of this disease and would like to avoid it at all costs. You can't avoid genetics, but there are various conditions and risks you might be putting on yourself that could leave you susceptible to this. If you notice yourself seeing these risks within you, it might be best to take action and eliminate these risks from your life as much as you can.

Risk Factors

There are two risk factors you can't change, and that is age and genetics. Whatever your parents passed to you is a genetic code that at this point can be manipulated to stop you from having tis. While there are scientists looking to explore the e concept of gene manipulation, it's not possible at this time. However, there is another major risk that you can control, and it's also linked to a whole slew of other major health conditions as well.

That risk factor is cardiovascular health. You've probably heard many expound on it, for it's one of the worst conditions to have. It's life-threatening, in that if you do suffer from a heart attack, there is a strong chance you might perish. However, it also feeds into brain and nerve health as well.

Your body is a network of vessels that nourish all the major organs in your body, including the brain. The vessels near the brain stem re actually some of the biggest vessels in the body, but even a vessel far away can still cause damage as well.

If a blood vessel is stopped, then you're depriving that area of the body of oxygen and blood, which are two key components for its vitality. When dementia sets in, often the brain cells have died off, and you can see it on various scans.

When one suffers from vascular dementia, this is even more apparent, because often, the reason why they have dementia is due to a stroke, which is when an artery leading to the brain is blocked. Furthermore, if you already have had a stroke once, further damaging your blood vessels can cause your dementia to progressively worsen as well.

If you suffer from cardiovascular disease, this cases your impairments to become worse. Often, this will change not only the state of your heart, but the state of other major organs as well.

While you can't protect the brain, you can protect the heart, which will in turn protect the brain. Not only does minding your cardiovascular health benefit your brain, but it also benefits your heart as well, since heart disease is one of the largest killers in the world, and many don't watch for this until they're severely at risk.

If you do believe you suffer from cardiovascular issues, there are activities you can do to rectify it. For example, you can quit smoking, which is one of the major causes of heart disease. However, you should also look at what you're eating as well, since sugars are a major player in this. If you do believe you need to watch this, you should consult your doctor to help you get an accurate reading of your blood pressure, cholesterol, and blood sugar

Along with talking to your doctor about that, you should also find out what sorts of activities you can engage in to change this. If your doctor says you're overweight, work to change that by eating the right foods and getting adequate exercise. Taking control of your heart health is certainly important, and it can save your life.

Heart conditions can lead to dementia, so it's the major risk factor you can control that you'll be able to rectify as needed. While you can't control genetics, this is certainly one point, which can be remedied in a positive manner.

Preventative factors

With dementia, you can also work to prevent it. Genetics can't be changed, but if you know you're predisposed to it, there are ways to prevent it from sneaking in. Heart health is intimately connected to brain health, which makes it one of the preventative factors in fighting dementia. However, when it comes to improving your heart health, there are a few activities you can do which in turn will also help you fight dementia.

Exercise is the first activity you can engage in, since physical exercise can reduce vascular dementia along with other forms of dementia. Not only that, it also works to strengthen the blood vessels, allowing you to protect your body against heart conditions as well.

Not only that however, but it can also help strengthen your brain cells, since your brain will be getting more blood and oxygen, which are the nutrients it requires. The ideal amount of exercise is thirty minutes a day five days a week, with three of the days being more strenuous exercise.

You don't have to run a marathon obviously, but ideally you should at least try to get thirty minutes of brisk walking in every day, and work to also keep your muscles toned up with lightweight training. If you don't want to run, there are other activities you can do as well, such as swimming or cycling. It especially becomes important the older you get.

The second component is your diet, which has a significant impact on the body. What you eat has an impact on your brain and it does on your heart as well, often much larger than we assume.

When we eat junk food, we're building up plaque on our walls, and with enough plaque built up, heart disease sets in. Not only that, from a nutritional standpoint it's also important as well. When you eat bad food, you're only feeding your brain carbs and empty calories, instead of noshing vitamins. Often, the brain becomes starved for nutrients due to a lack of proper diet. However, this can be rectified by what you eat

The first course of action to take is to change your eating habits. Strive to incorporate more veggies into your diet, inducing eating them with various meats. You should go towards learner meats and avoid meats with a large amount of saturated fat, working to avoid trans fats as well. There are many healthy fats out there, such as nuts and shellfish, so pair those with other foods in your diet.

You should also work to avoid carbs. Carbs are bad for you, and often they lead to other health issues including diabetes and cardiovascular disease. So watch what you eat, because you never know what the food you eat could eventually lead to.

This chapter went over the risk factors and ways to prevent this condition from coming about in your life. Take heed to these, and watch what you eat, so you can have a healthier, happier body.

Conclusion

Thank you again for downloading this book!

I hope this book was able to help you to understand all about dementia. Dementia is a condition that can be very hard for those living around the person to cope with, and for those affected, it can really put a damper on their life. However, it's a disease that can be treated, but ultimately, while there isn't a cure, there is a way to deal with those that are afflicted by this, and I hope that this book was able to give you a sort of understanding on how dementia affects those around people, how one can treat those that suffer from it, and the various facets of this condition.

The next step is to help those that suffer from that condition. Further understanding this is essential to the success of coping with this. Often, if a person does start to notice they're afflicted with this, they should seek help for their condition. If you know of someone around that's suffering from this, you should do what's best for him or her, and take him or her to a medical professional. It's quite the situation to face, but often, for those that are affected by it, early detection can lead to better treatment, and it can help to minimize or hinder the effects for a certain period of time as well.

Thank you and good luck!